Restful Nights:

Navigating the Science and Solutions of Sleep

By

Hugh Mclaughlan

Welcome to "Restful Nights: Navigating the Science and Solutions of Sleep." In the quiet moments between dusk and dawn, we all seek the elusive embrace of restful slumber. This book is an exploration into the profound realm of sleep—the science that governs it and the practical solutions that pave the way to rejuvenating nights. Join me on a journey through the mysteries of the night, as we unravel the complexities of sleep and discover the keys to unlocking peaceful, restorative rest. In a world that often moves at a relentless pace, let's embark on a quest for nights that not only harbour dreams but also provide the foundation for vibrant, waking days.

Contents

Introduction

Welcome to "Restful Nights: Navigating the Science and Solutions of Sleep," a journey into the profound world of slumber and its impact on our physical, mental, and emotional well-being. In the hustle and bustle of our modern lives, the importance of quality sleep often takes a back seat. This book seeks to illuminate the vital role that sleep plays in our lives, inviting you to explore the fascinating science behind it and discover practical solutions for achieving restful nights.

The nocturnal odyssey begins with an exploration of the intricacies of sleep, unveiling the stages, rhythms, and physiological wonders that unfold when we close our eyes. We'll delve into the science that governs our nightly rest, examining the profound effects sleep has on our overall health. As we journey further, we'll confront common sleep challenges, from the persistent grip of insomnia to the subtle disturbances of restless leg syndrome, offering insights and strategies to overcome these obstacles.

Amidst the scientific exploration, this book is also a guide to practical wisdom. From creating a sleep-friendly environment to developing consistent bedtime routines, we'll uncover actionable tips to enhance the quality of your sleep. Along the way, we'll tackle the intricate interplay between sleep and mental health, addressing the impact of stress, anxiety, and sleep disorders on our nightly repose. Join me on this adventure through the land of dreams and wakefulness, where the mysteries of the night unfold, and the keys to a more vibrant, rested life await.

The importance of sleep

Sleep is not merely a nightly pause in our busy lives; it is a fundamental pillar of our overall well-being. In the realm of physical health, sleep plays a crucial role in the restoration and repair of various bodily functions. It is during the restful phases of sleep that our immune system strengthens, hormones rebalance, and tissues undergo essential repair processes. Furthermore, adequate sleep is linked to improved cardiovascular health, better metabolism, and an overall reduced risk of chronic diseases.

Equally significant is the impact of sleep on mental health. The night's repose is a period of cognitive regeneration, where memories are consolidated, and the brain processes emotions experienced throughout the day. Insufficient sleep has been linked to heightened stress levels, anxiety, and an increased susceptibility to mood disorders. Conversely, a well-rested mind is better equipped to handle challenges, make sound decisions, and maintain emotional resilience.

Beyond the individual benefits, the importance of sleep extends to societal well-being. Sleep deficiency has been associated with impaired cognitive function, decreased productivity, and an increased risk of accidents. In a world that values constant productivity and connectivity, recognising the pivotal role of sleep is essential for fostering a healthier and more vibrant global community. By appreciating and prioritising the significance of quality sleep, we pave the way for individuals to lead more fulfilling lives and contribute meaningfully to the world around them.

In the labyrinth of shift work, my struggle with sleep emerged as an insidious adversary. The irregular hours and constant shift changes disrupted the delicate balance my body had known. Nights blended into days, and as my circadian rhythm faltered, so did the sanctuary of rest. Initially, the fatigue seemed manageable, a mere consequence of the job's demands. However, the toll on my sleep began to cast shadows on both my mental and physical well-being.

The relentless battle against sleep deprivation became a silent war waged beneath the surface of my waking hours. As the quality of my sleep diminished, so did my ability to focus and make sound decisions during my shifts. The fog of exhaustion clouded my mind, creating a mental strain that intensified with each passing day. The cognitive toll was palpable – a once-sharp mind dulled by the constant struggle to find rest in the disjointed cadence of my work hours.

Physically, the toll was equally profound. The irregular sleep patterns took a toll on my body's natural rhythms. I felt the weariness settling into my bones, a persistent ache that seemed to echo the disarray of my disrupted sleep schedule. The lack of consistent rest impacted my immune system, making me more susceptible to illnesses. The physical fatigue became an unwelcome companion, eroding my resilience and diminishing my overall health.

Beyond the tangible effects, the emotional toll of battling sleep deprivation became increasingly apparent. The constant exhaustion gave rise to heightened stress levels and mood swings. The wear and tear on my mental health manifested in moments of frustration, irritability, and an overwhelming sense of fatigue-induced despair. The once-reliable coping mechanisms seemed insufficient against the relentless strain on my mind and body.

In the crucible of shift work, the struggle against sleep deprivation has become an arduous journey with far-reaching implications. The impact on both mental and physical health serves as a poignant reminder of the critical need for adequate sleep. As I navigate the challenges of this demanding schedule, finding strategies to prioritise and improve my sleep has become a vital pursuit, a beacon of hope in the quest for restored well-being amidst the tumultuous seas of shift work.

In the quest for respite from the relentless battle against sleep disruption in my shift work, I turned to meditation and hypnotherapy as beacons of solace. Intrigued by the promise of calming the storm within my mind, I embarked on a journey of mindfulness and subconscious exploration.

Meditation became my daily ritual, a sanctuary amid the chaos. Through guided breathing and focused awareness, I sought refuge from the relentless demands of my work hours. In those moments of stillness, I discovered a profound sense of peace. The practice not only became a respite for my mind but also a beacon guiding me towards better sleep. Each session acted as a balm, gradually easing the strain and fostering a mental clarity that eluded me in the chaotic wakefulness of my shift work.

Hypnotherapy, with its exploration of the subconscious, became another avenue in my pursuit of restful nights. Guided by a therapist, I delved into the depths of my mind, addressing the underlying anxieties and patterns that sabotaged my sleep. The process was a revelation, unearthing buried stressors and gently coaxing my subconscious towards a state of calm. Through hypnotherapy, I began to rewrite the narrative of my sleep, unraveling the knots that had tightened over countless sleepless nights.

Together, meditation and hypnotherapy acted as a dynamic duo in my battle against sleep disruption. The mindfulness cultivated through meditation served as a shield against the relentless onslaught of stress, allowing me to navigate the challenges of shift work with greater resilience. Hypnotherapy, on the other hand, became a lantern illuminating the hidden corridors of my subconscious, unraveling the intricate web of thoughts that hindered rest.

While the journey is ongoing, the integration of these practices into my routine has marked a transformative chapter. Meditation and hypnotherapy, in their unique ways, have provided me with tools to reclaim my sleep and foster a mindset that embraces rest amidst the unpredictable rhythm of shift work. As I continue to explore the depths of mindfulness and subconscious healing, I find solace in the hope that each session brings me one step closer to the elusive embrace of a truly restful night.

Overview of this Book

"Restful Nights: Navigating the Science and Solutions of Sleep" is a comprehensive guide that transcends the ordinary boundaries of sleep literature. In the opening chapters, we embark on a fascinating exploration of the science behind sleep. Unveiling the intricate stages, circadian rhythms, and the profound physiological processes that occur during rest, readers will gain a deep understanding of the mechanics governing our nightly repose. The book establishes a foundation by highlighting the critical role sleep plays in our physical health, from immune system fortification to the repair of vital bodily functions, setting the stage for a holistic understanding of the sleep experience.

As we venture further into the pages, the narrative shifts to address common sleep challenges that many individuals encounter. From the relentless grip of insomnia to the nuanced disturbances of conditions like sleep apnea and restless leg syndrome, the book offers insights and strategies to navigate these obstacles. This practical wisdom extends into the heart of the book, where readers discover actionable tips for achieving better sleep. From creating a sleep-conducive environment to establishing consistent bedtime routines, the guide provides tangible solutions for enhancing the quality of nightly rest, emphasising the tangible impact on overall health and well-being.

However, "Restful Nights" is not solely a scientific or practical manual. It's an immersive experience that explores the intimate connection between sleep and mental health. Addressing the profound impact of stress, anxiety, and various sleep disorders, the book delves into the intricate interplay between the mind and nightly repose. The journey concludes with a reflection on the broader societal implications of prioritising quality sleep, recognising its role in fostering cognitive function, productivity, and overall community well-being. "Restful Nights" is not just a guide to better sleep; it is an invitation to unlock the secrets of the night and embrace a more vibrant, rested life.

The Science of Sleep

Welcome to the captivating realm of the science of sleep, where each night unfolds a symphony of physiological processes that intricately orchestrate our restorative journey. In this exploration, we peel back the layers of the nocturnal world, revealing the stages, rhythms, and fascinating intricacies that characterise our nightly repose. The journey commences with an exploration of sleep stages—each offering a unique choreography of brain activity, from the initial descent into light sleep to the profound depths of rapid eye movement (REM) sleep, where dreams come to life. Understanding these stages provides a foundation for unraveling the mysterious dance that transpires within us as we traverse the landscape of the night.

As we venture deeper into the science of sleep, we encounter the rhythmic heartbeat of our internal clock—the circadian rhythm. This innate biological rhythm governs the ebb and flow of various bodily functions, orchestrating a symphony of hormonal releases and metabolic shifts to synchronise with the external world. Delving into the circadian rhythm offers insights into the optimal times for sleep and wakefulness, providing a roadmap for aligning our daily lives with the natural cadence that our bodies crave.

The science of sleep is not confined to the internal workings of our bodies; it extends its tendrils into the vast tapestry of physical and mental health. From immune system rejuvenation to memory consolidation, we unravel the profound ways in which sleep contributes to overall well-being. Join me in this enlightening journey through the science of sleep, where we uncover the mysteries that unfold when we surrender to the embrace of the night.

Stages of Sleep

Understanding the Stages of Sleep

Embarking on the exploration of sleep necessitates a nuanced understanding of its various stages, each contributing to the complex tapestry of nocturnal rejuvenation. These stages, collectively known as the sleep cycle, are characterised by distinct patterns of brain activity and physiological changes. The sleep cycle is divided into two main categories: Non-Rapid Eye Movement (NREM) sleep and Rapid Eye Movement (REM) sleep.

NREM Stage 1 (N1): The Gateway to Sleep

- This initial stage marks the transition from wakefulness to sleep. Lasting for a brief period, N1 is a light sleep stage where individuals can be easily awakened. Muscle activity decreases, and the first inklings of relaxation set in. This stage serves as a gateway to the deeper realms of sleep.

NREM Stage 2 (N2): Light Sleep

- N2 is a slightly deeper stage characterised by the onset of true sleep. During this phase, heart rate and body temperature decrease, and the body prepares for more profound rest. Sleep spindles—brief bursts of brain activity—begin to emerge, contributing to the overall stabilisation of sleep.

NREM Stage 3 (N3): Deep Sleep

- N3, often referred to as slow-wave sleep (SWS) or deep sleep, is the stage where the body undergoes essential restoration and repair. It is during this phase that growth hormone is released, contributing to physical rejuvenation. N3 is particularly crucial for overall well-being, and disturbances in this deep sleep stage can impact various bodily functions.

Rapid Eye Movement (REM) Sleep: The Dreaming Stage

- REM sleep is a distinctive stage marked by rapid eye movements, increased brain activity, and vivid dreams. Despite the heightened brain activity, the voluntary muscles become temporarily paralysed, preventing individuals from acting out their dreams. REM sleep plays a vital role in cognitive processes, emotion regulation, and memory consolidation, contributing to mental and emotional well-being.

Understanding these stages is foundational to unraveling the intricacies of sleep, providing valuable insights into the nightly voyage that our minds and bodies undertake. As we delve deeper into the subsequent chapters, we'll uncover the significance of each stage and its profound impact on our overall health.

Quote

"In the dance of dreams, our minds choreograph a symphony through the stages of sleep, where each slumbering moment whispers the untold stories of our subconscious existence."

Circadian Rhythms

The Harmonious Dance of Circadian Rhythms

Central to the orchestration of our daily lives is the mesmerising cadence of circadian rhythms, an internal timekeeping system that synchronises with the external world. These rhythms, often referred to as the body's biological clock, regulate various physiological processes over a roughly 24-hour cycle. The master conductor of this intricate symphony is the suprachiasmatic nucleus (SCN) in the brain, responding to external cues like light to maintain harmony within the body's internal environment.

The Daily Ebb and Flow: Understanding Circadian Phases

Circadian rhythms manifest in distinct phases, influencing our energy levels, mood, and cognitive performance. The wakefulness-promoting hormone cortisol peaks in the early morning, heralding the start of the active phase. As the day unfolds, body temperature rises, contributing to heightened alertness. Evening signals a shift towards the restful phase, with melatonin secretion rising, preparing the body for sleep. This rhythmic ebb and flow reflects the adaptive nature of our biological clock, finely tuned to optimise functioning across various activities throughout the day.

The Impact of Modern Lifestyles: Circadian Disruptions

In today's fast-paced world, circadian rhythms can face disruptions due to factors such as irregular sleep schedules, exposure to artificial light at night, and shift work. These disruptions can lead to desynchronisation, impacting sleep quality, mood, and overall health. Understanding the delicate balance of circadian rhythms becomes paramount in mitigating these challenges, emphasising the importance of aligning daily activities with the body's natural clock for optimal well-being.

Circadian Rhythms and Sleep: A Symbiotic
Relationship

Circadian rhythms and sleep are intricately entwined, influencing one another in a symbiotic dance. Sleep-wake cycles, hormone release, and even cognitive function are governed by the body's internal clock. Acknowledging this relationship becomes essential in fostering healthy sleep habits and overall wellness. In the chapters to come, we'll explore how circadian rhythms contribute not only to the science of sleep but also to our holistic understanding of well-being, guiding us towards a more harmonious integration of rest and wakefulness in our lives.

Quote

"In the rhythmic dance of time, our circadian clock
orchestrates the harmony of life – a synchronised
melody that guides our energy, sleep, and vitality,
revealing the beauty of balance in the cadence of
existence."

Roles of sleep in physical and mental health

The Vital Role of Sleep in Physical Health

Quality sleep is a cornerstone of physical health, providing the body with a crucial opportunity for restoration and repair. During deep sleep stages, such as slow-wave sleep (SWS), the body releases growth hormone, facilitating the mending of tissues, muscles, and bones. Furthermore, the immune system strengthens during sleep, enhancing its ability to defend against infections and illnesses. The profound impact of sleep on physical health extends beyond mere rejuvenation, contributing to overall resilience and vitality.

Cognitive Rejuvenation: The Mental Health Connection

Inextricably linked to physical health, the role of sleep in mental well-being is equally significant. Sleep is a dynamic process that actively contributes to cognitive functions, including memory consolidation, learning, and problem-solving. The various stages of sleep play distinct roles in these mental processes, ensuring that our brains are not only well-rested but also adept at processing and storing information. Inadequate sleep has been associated with cognitive impairments, difficulty concentrating, and increased susceptibility to mood disorders.

Emotional Balance and Sleep Quality

The emotional landscape is intricately tied to the quality of our sleep. Adequate sleep fosters emotional resilience, allowing individuals to navigate stressors more effectively. Conversely, chronic sleep deprivation or sleep disorders can exacerbate emotional challenges, contributing to increased irritability, anxiety, and heightened emotional reactivity. Recognising the symbiotic relationship between sleep and emotional well-being underscores the importance of prioritising rest for overall mental health.

The Impact of Sleep on Stress Hormones

Sleep plays a pivotal role in regulating stress hormones, such as cortisol. Adequate sleep helps maintain a balanced cortisol rhythm, ensuring it peaks in the early morning to promote wakefulness and gradually decreases throughout the day. Disruptions in this rhythm due to inadequate sleep or irregular sleep patterns can contribute to heightened stress levels, potentially leading to long-term negative impacts on both physical and mental health.

A Comprehensive Approach to Well-being

In the tapestry of overall health, sleep is not a passive state but an active contributor to our well-being. Recognising the intricate interplay between physical and mental health positions sleep as a cornerstone of a holistic approach to self-care. The subsequent chapters of this book will further illuminate the ways in which prioritising and optimising sleep can lead to enhanced physical and mental resilience, fostering a more vibrant and fulfilling life.

Quotes

"In the silent embrace of sleep, our bodies mend, minds rejuvenate, and the symphony of well-being unfolds – for in the dance between rest and wakefulness, health finds its greatest ally, and the soul replenishes its resilience."

"Sleep, the quiet architect of vitality, shapes our physical strength and fortifies the fortress of mental resilience. In the realm of dreams, our bodies heal, minds renew, and the essence of true health emerges, painting a canvas of well-being with each peaceful slumber."

Winston Churchill once remarked, "Nature has not intended mankind to work from eight in the morning until midnight without that refreshment of blessed oblivion which, even if it only lasts twenty minutes, is sufficient to renew all the vital forces." His words underline the importance of sleep in maintaining mental well-being and the rejuvenation it brings to our essential energies.

Common sleep challenges

Insomnia: The Elusive Embrace of Sleep

Insomnia, a prevalent sleep challenge, manifests as persistent difficulty falling or staying asleep. This multifaceted condition often results from a combination of factors such as stress, anxiety, or disrupted sleep routines. Chronic insomnia can lead to daytime fatigue, diminished cognitive function, and an overall decline in quality of life. Exploring strategies to address the root causes and promote healthy sleep habits is essential for those grappling with this elusive embrace of rest.

Sleep Apnea: A Breath Interrupted

Sleep apnea disrupts the natural breathing pattern during sleep, characterised by pauses in breathing and subsequent awakenings. The most common type, obstructive sleep apnea, occurs when the airway is partially or fully blocked. This condition not only compromises sleep quality but can also contribute to cardiovascular issues and heightened daytime sleepiness. Management often involves lifestyle changes, the use of continuous positive airway pressure (CPAP) devices, or other interventions to improve airflow.

Restless Leg Syndrome: The Dance of Discomfort

Restless Leg Syndrome (RLS) introduces a peculiar dance of discomfort during sleep, characterised by an irresistible urge to move the legs. This condition often intensifies in the evening or at night, disrupting the ability to settle into restful sleep. Understanding lifestyle factors, incorporating relaxation techniques, and, in some cases, medication can mitigate the symptoms and bring relief to those contending with the restless leg's nocturnal rhythm.

Addressing Stress and Anxiety: The Sleep Disruptors

Stress and anxiety, pervasive challenges in modern life, cast a long shadow on the tranquility of sleep. The hyperarousal caused by persistent stress or anxiety can make it challenging to transition into a restful state. Establishing stress management techniques, such as mindfulness or relaxation exercises, can be instrumental in mitigating these disruptions, creating a more conducive environment for peaceful slumber.

Circadian Rhythm Disorders: Navigating Time's Influence

Circadian rhythm disorders, encompassing conditions like delayed sleep phase syndrome or shift work disorder, highlight the impact of our internal clock on sleep patterns. Disruptions to the natural circadian rhythm can lead to difficulty falling asleep at desired times or maintaining consistent sleep-wake cycles. Strategies involve adjusting sleep schedules, optimising sleep environments, and incorporating light exposure to align the body's internal clock with external demands.

Narcolepsy: Navigating Unpredictable Sleepiness

Narcolepsy, a neurological disorder, introduces uncontrollable bouts of daytime sleepiness, often accompanied by sudden muscle weakness (cataplexy). This condition can profoundly affect daily functioning and quality of life. While there is no cure, medications and lifestyle adjustments can help manage symptoms, allowing individuals with narcolepsy to navigate the delicate balance between wakefulness and the unpredictable allure of sleep.

Parasomnias: Intricacies of Sleep-Related Behaviours

Parasomnias encompass a variety of abnormal behaviours or movements during sleep. This category includes phenomena like sleepwalking, night terrors, and sleep-related eating disorder. These behaviours can disrupt sleep continuity and lead to safety concerns. Understanding triggers and implementing safety measures in the sleep environment are crucial aspects of managing parasomnias.

Periodic Limb Movement Disorder (PLMD): The Rhythmic Stirrings

PLMD involves repetitive movements, usually in the legs, during sleep. These rhythmic movements can disrupt sleep, leading to frequent awakenings and subsequent daytime fatigue. Identifying potential underlying causes, such as iron deficiency, and exploring therapeutic interventions can be instrumental in alleviating symptoms and improving sleep quality.

Understanding these common sleep challenges provides a roadmap for individuals seeking solutions to enhance their sleep quality and overall well-being. In the following chapters, we'll delve into specific strategies and insights to address these challenges, fostering a more harmonious relationship with the night and the restorative embrace of sleep.

Each sleep challenge presents a unique set of circumstances and considerations, often requiring a tailored approach for effective management. Addressing these challenges involves a combination of lifestyle modifications, behavioural strategies, and, in some cases, medical interventions. As we delve into specific topics in the subsequent chapters, we'll further explore the intricacies of these challenges and provide insights to empower individuals in their quest for restful nights.

Quote

"In the quiet hours of night, common sleep challenges echo through the darkness, but within each struggle lies the potential for understanding, adaptation, and the dawning light of restful resilience."

Bill Gates has also shared insights on sleep challenges, stating, "I used to pull all-nighters to get ahead, but I've since learned that sacrificing sleep is a poor way to accomplish anything. Sleep deprivation impairs our ability to make decisions and be creative, ultimately hindering success rather than propelling it." Gates emphasises the negative impact of sleep deprivation on decision-making and creativity, urging the importance of addressing sleep challenges for optimal performance.

Practical tips for better sleep

Creating a Sleep-Friendly Environment: The Sanctuary of Serenity

Establishing a serene sleep environment is foundational to better sleep. This involves keeping the bedroom cool, dark, and quiet. Consider investing in blackout curtains, using earplugs, or employing white noise machines to minimise disturbances. Selecting a comfortable mattress and pillows that support your preferred sleeping position contributes to a restful sleep sanctuary.

Developing a Consistent Sleep Routine: The Power of Predictability

Crafting a consistent sleep routine signals to your body that it's time to wind down. Establish a regular bedtime and wake-up time, even on weekends, to regulate your internal clock. Engage in calming activities before bed, such as reading a book, taking a warm bath, or practicing relaxation techniques. Consistency reinforces your body's natural circadian rhythm, enhancing the predictability of sleep.

Limiting Exposure to Screens: Dimming the Digital Glow

The blue light emitted by screens can interfere with the production of melatonin, the hormone that regulates sleep. Aim to reduce screen time at least an hour before bedtime. Consider using "night mode" on devices or wearing blue light-blocking glasses to mitigate the impact of screens on your circadian rhythm.

Monitoring Caffeine and Alcohol Intake: Balancing Beverages

Caffeine and alcohol can disrupt sleep patterns. Limit the intake of caffeinated beverages in the afternoon and evening, and be mindful of the sedative effects of alcohol, which can initially induce drowsiness but later interfere with the deeper stages of sleep. Hydrate with water instead, particularly in the hours leading up to bedtime.

Regular Exercise: Energising the Body for Sleep

Incorporating regular physical activity into your routine can promote better sleep. Engage in moderate exercise, such as walking or yoga, earlier in the day to reap the benefits without overstimulating the body close to bedtime. Regular exercise contributes to overall well-being, reducing stress and anxiety that may interfere with sleep.

Mindful Nutrition: Nourishing for the Night

Be mindful of your eating habits, especially in the evening. Avoid heavy meals close to bedtime, as digestion can disrupt sleep. Opt for a light, balanced snack if hunger strikes before bedtime. Consider foods rich in tryptophan, such as turkey or nuts, which can support the production of sleep-inducing serotonin.

Mindfulness and Relaxation Techniques: Calming the Mind

Incorporating mindfulness and relaxation practices into your bedtime routine can help quiet the mind and prepare it for rest. Techniques such as deep breathing exercises, progressive muscle relaxation, or guided imagery can be effective in reducing stress and promoting a sense of calm before sleep.

Establishing a Technology Curfew: Unplugging for Rest

Create a technology curfew by powering down electronic devices at least an hour before bedtime. The blue light emitted from screens can suppress melatonin production, making it harder to fall asleep. Disconnecting from screens allows your brain to transition into a more relaxed state conducive to sleep.

Optimising Nap Habits: A Brief Siesta Strategy

If you find yourself needing a nap during the day, keep it short and early. A brief nap of 20-30 minutes can provide a quick energy boost without interfering with nighttime sleep. Avoid napping too close to bedtime, as it may disrupt your ability to fall asleep at night.

Journaling: Unloading Thoughts Before Bed

Consider keeping a journal to jot down thoughts, concerns, or reflections before bedtime. This practice helps unload your mind and prevents overthinking as you try to fall asleep. It can be a therapeutic way to release the day's stressors and promote mental clarity for a more restful night.

Temperature Regulation: Cool Comfort for Sleep

Maintain a comfortable room temperature conducive to sleep. The ideal bedroom temperature is generally between 60-67 degrees Fahrenheit (15-20 degrees Celsius). Experiment with bedding layers to find the right combination that keeps you comfortably cool throughout the night.

Seeking Professional Help: Consulting Sleep Experts

If persistent sleep challenges persist, seeking guidance from healthcare professionals or sleep specialists is essential. They can conduct assessments, such as sleep studies, to identify underlying sleep disorders or offer personalised advice based on your unique sleep patterns and challenges.

Incorporating these tips into your daily routine fosters a sleep-friendly lifestyle, enhancing the quality of your nightly rest. Experiment with these strategies, and tailor them to your preferences to create a personalised approach to better sleep. As we explore these tips in greater detail in the following chapters, you'll gain a deeper understanding of how each element contributes to the art of restful nights.

Quote

"In the gentle embrace of a good night's sleep, let mindful moments be the lullabies that guide you. From soothing routines to peaceful thoughts, the tips for better sleep weave a tapestry of rest, where each thread creates a sanctuary for dreams to flourish and vitality to awaken."

Oprah Winfrey advocates for quality sleep, stating, "Create a sacred bedtime ritual. Disconnect from the day, release worries, and immerse yourself in a calming routine. Whether it's reading, gentle stretching, or deep-breathing exercises, these intentional moments before sleep can be transformative, nurturing a restful night that echoes into a vibrant tomorrow."

The distinction between a sleep disorder and a sleep challenge lies in the severity, persistence, and impact on one's overall well-being. A sleep challenge often refers to occasional difficulties in achieving or maintaining quality sleep, which may be influenced by lifestyle factors, stress, or temporary disruptions. These challenges are common and can often be addressed through changes in sleep hygiene or daily routines. On the other hand, a sleep disorder involves more persistent and clinically significant disruptions to sleep patterns. These disorders, such as insomnia, sleep apnea, or narcolepsy, often require professional intervention for accurate diagnosis and management. While sleep challenges may be managed with lifestyle adjustments, a sleep disorder may necessitate a more comprehensive approach, involving medical evaluation, specialised treatments, or interventions tailored to the specific disorder.

The causes of sleep disorders are multifaceted, often arising from a complex interplay of biological, psychological, and environmental factors. In the case of insomnia, stress and anxiety are common culprits, contributing to persistent difficulties in falling or staying asleep. Lifestyle factors, irregular sleep schedules, or disruptions in circadian rhythms can further exacerbate insomnia. Additionally, underlying medical conditions, such as depression or chronic pain, may contribute to this sleep disorder. Understanding and addressing the root causes, whether they be lifestyle-related or stemming from mental health concerns, is essential in developing effective strategies for managing insomnia.

Sleep apnea is frequently linked to structural issues in the airway that lead to repeated partial or complete blockages during sleep. Obesity, which can contribute to the narrowing of the airway, is a significant risk factor. Other causes include genetic predispositions, anatomical abnormalities, or conditions that affect muscle tone, such as hypothyroidism. Narcolepsy, on the other hand, is thought to be associated with an imbalance in neurotransmitters in the brain, particularly hypocretin. This deficiency may be the result of genetic factors or autoimmune processes. Identifying and addressing these specific causes, be they related to anatomy, genetics, or neurochemistry, is crucial for tailoring effective treatments and management strategies for sleep disorders.

Insomnia: The Persistent Struggle for Sleep

Insomnia, one of the most prevalent sleep disorders, manifests as difficulty falling asleep or staying asleep, leading to inadequate or non-restorative sleep. Persistent insomnia can be caused by various factors, including stress, anxiety, or underlying medical conditions. Individuals with insomnia often experience daytime fatigue, impaired concentration, and mood disturbances, impacting both their mental and physical well-being.

Sleep Apnea: Interrupted Breathing, Disrupted Sleep

Sleep apnea is characterised by recurrent interruptions in breathing during sleep, often due to the partial or complete collapse of the upper airway. These pauses, known as apneas, trigger brief awakenings, preventing individuals from reaching deeper, more restful stages of sleep. Beyond the immediate impact on sleep quality, untreated sleep apnea is associated with an increased risk of cardiovascular issues, including hypertension and heart disease.

Narcolepsy: Uncontrollable Sleepiness and Cataplexy

Narcolepsy is a neurological disorder characterised by excessive daytime sleepiness, often leading to uncontrollable episodes of falling asleep during daily activities. Additionally, individuals with narcolepsy may experience cataplexy, a sudden loss of muscle tone triggered by strong emotions. This disorder significantly affects daily functioning, requiring tailored treatments, such as medications and lifestyle adjustments, to manage symptoms effectively.

Restless Leg Syndrome (RLS): The Disruptive Urge to Move

Restless Leg Syndrome is characterised by an irresistible urge to move the legs, often accompanied by uncomfortable sensations, particularly in the evening or at night. These sensations can interfere with the ability to relax and fall asleep. RLS disrupts sleep continuity, leading to sleep fragmentation and daytime fatigue. Identifying triggers and incorporating lifestyle changes are integral components of managing this condition.

Parasomnias: Unusual Behaviours During Sleep

Parasomnias encompass a variety of abnormal behaviours or movements during sleep. Sleepwalking, night terrors, and sleep-related eating disorders are examples of parasomnias that can disrupt sleep and pose safety concerns. These phenomena often arise during specific sleep stages and may require a combination of environmental adjustments and, in some cases, medical intervention to manage effectively.

Circadian Rhythm Sleep Disorders:

These disorders involve a misalignment between the internal circadian clock and the desired sleep-wake schedule. Conditions like delayed sleep phase syndrome, where individuals have a later-than-desired sleep onset, or shift work sleep disorder, common among those with irregular work hours, fall under this category. Treatment often involves aligning sleep schedules with the natural circadian rhythm through behavioural and environmental adjustments.

Periodic Limb Movement Disorder (PLMD):

PLMD is characterised by repetitive limb movements, usually involving the legs, during sleep. These movements can lead to frequent awakenings, disrupting the overall quality of sleep. PLMD is often associated with conditions like restless leg syndrome and may require interventions such as medication or lifestyle adjustments to alleviate symptoms.

Sleep-Related Eating Disorder (SRED):

SRED involves the consumption of food during partial arousal from sleep, often leading to overeating and sometimes harmful behaviours such as cooking or consuming non-food items. This parasomnia can impact both sleep quality and overall health and may require a combination of behavioural therapy and medical intervention for effective management.

Nightmare Disorder:

While occasional nightmares are normal, recurrent and distressing nightmares can be classified as a sleep disorder. Nightmare disorder may be linked to various factors, including stress, trauma, or certain medications. Addressing underlying psychological factors through therapy and creating a sleep-friendly environment can help manage this disorder.

Understanding and addressing sleep disorders involve a comprehensive approach, including medical evaluation, lifestyle modifications, and, when necessary, specialised treatments. If persistent sleep issues are suspected, seeking guidance from healthcare professionals or sleep specialists is crucial for accurate diagnosis and the development of an effective management plan tailored to individual needs.

Seeking help with sleep disorders

Seeking help for sleep disorders is a crucial step toward improving overall well-being and addressing the specific challenges disrupting one's sleep. The journey often begins with consulting a healthcare professional, such as a primary care physician or a sleep specialist, who can conduct a comprehensive evaluation. This evaluation may involve discussing the individual's sleep history, daily routines, and any potential underlying health conditions or stressors contributing to the sleep disorder. The information gathered during this process helps in identifying the specific nature of the sleep issue and guides the development of an appropriate treatment plan.

A healthcare professional may recommend a sleep study, also known as polysomnography, to monitor various physiological parameters during sleep. This diagnostic tool helps to identify patterns and abnormalities in sleep architecture, assisting in the accurate diagnosis of sleep disorders. Sleep studies can be conducted in a sleep centre or, in some cases, at home with portable monitoring devices. The results provide valuable insights into factors such as breathing patterns, brain activity, and limb movements during sleep.

Treatment approaches for sleep disorders vary based on the specific diagnosis. You Lifestyle modifications, such as improving sleep hygiene or adjusting daily routines, are often recommended. Behavioural therapies, including cognitive-behavioural therapy for insomnia (CBT-I), can be effective in addressing certain sleep disorders. In cases where medical interventions are necessary, medications or devices may be prescribed to manage symptoms. Ongoing communication with healthcare providers is vital to monitor progress, adjust treatment plans as needed, and ensure comprehensive care for individuals seeking help with sleep disorders.

Beyond medical professionals, support groups and mental health professionals can play integral roles in the journey to better sleep. Sharing experiences with others who face similar challenges can provide emotional support and practical insights. Mental health professionals, such as psychologists or counsellors, can assist in addressing underlying psychological factors contributing to sleep disorders, offering strategies to manage stress, anxiety, or other issues affecting sleep. Seeking help is not only a path to improved sleep but also a commitment to overall health and quality of life.

Sleep Disorder Treatment Options

Lifestyle Modifications: Foundational Changes for Better Sleep

For many sleep disorders, lifestyle modifications serve as a primary and often foundational component of treatment. This includes establishing consistent sleep routines, creating a sleep-conducive environment, and adopting healthy sleep hygiene practices. Lifestyle adjustments may also involve managing stress through relaxation techniques, regular exercise, and maintaining a balanced diet. These changes aim to promote overall well-being and set the stage for improved sleep.

Behavioural Therapies: Targeting Cognitive Patterns

Behavioural therapies, such as Cognitive-Behavioural Therapy for Insomnia (CBT-I), are evidence-based approaches that address the cognitive and behavioural patterns contributing to sleep disorders. CBT-I focuses on modifying thoughts and behaviours that hinder sleep, offering strategies to overcome insomnia. This therapeutic approach aims to break the cycle of negative sleep-related thoughts and establish healthier associations with bedtime and sleep.

Medications: Pharmacological Support for Symptom Management

Pharmacological interventions are often considered for certain sleep disorders, particularly when lifestyle changes and behavioural therapies prove insufficient. Medications may include sleep aids, such as benzodiazepines or non-benzodiazepine hypnotics, to induce sleep or manage insomnia. For sleep disorders like sleep apnea, continuous positive airway pressure (CPAP) machines are commonly prescribed to maintain open airways during sleep.

CPAP and Other Devices: Mechanical Support for Sleep Apnea

Continuous Positive Airway Pressure (CPAP) devices are a cornerstone in managing sleep apnea. These machines deliver a continuous stream of air, preventing airway collapse during sleep. Other devices, such as dental appliances, may be recommended based on individual needs and the specific characteristics of sleep apnea. Customised to each patient, these devices provide mechanical support to alleviate breathing issues and enhance sleep quality.

Light Therapy: Regulating Circadian Rhythms

Light therapy is often utilised to manage circadian rhythm disorders, such as delayed sleep phase syndrome or shift work sleep disorder. This treatment involves exposure to bright light, typically in the morning, to regulate the body's internal clock. Light therapy can help reset circadian rhythms, promoting alertness during waking hours and enhancing the ability to sleep at desired times.

Surgical Interventions: Addressing Structural Issues

For sleep disorders with underlying structural issues, surgical interventions may be considered. Surgical options are often explored in cases of sleep apnea where anatomical factors contribute to airway obstruction. Procedures such as uvulopalatopharyngoplasty (UPPP) or genioglossus advancement (GA) aim to alleviate blockages and improve airflow during sleep. Surgical interventions are typically reserved for cases where other treatments have proven ineffective or impractical.

Treatment plans are highly individualised, taking into account the specific nature of the sleep disorder, its underlying causes, and the patient's overall health. Consultation with healthcare professionals, including sleep specialists, is crucial to determine the most appropriate combination of treatments tailored to address the unique challenges of each individual's sleep disorder.

Melatonin Supplements: Regulating Sleep-Wake Cycles

Melatonin supplements are commonly used to address circadian rhythm disorders or jet lag. Melatonin is a hormone that plays a key role in regulating sleep-wake cycles. Supplemental melatonin can help signal to the body that it's time to sleep, making it beneficial for individuals struggling with disrupted sleep patterns.

Dental Devices: Managing Snoring and Mild Sleep Apnea

Dental devices, such as mandibular advancement devices (MADs) or tongue-retaining devices, may be recommended to manage snoring and mild to moderate sleep apnea. These devices work by repositioning the jaw or tongue to keep the airway open during sleep, reducing the likelihood of airway collapse.

Weight Management: Addressing Obesity-Related Sleep Apnea

For individuals with sleep apnea linked to obesity, weight management becomes a crucial aspect of treatment. Losing excess weight can alleviate pressure on the airway, reducing the severity of sleep apnea symptoms. Lifestyle changes, including dietary modifications and regular exercise, are often recommended in conjunction with other treatments.

Biofeedback and Relaxation Techniques: Stress Reduction for Better Sleep

Biofeedback and relaxation techniques, such as progressive muscle relaxation or biofeedback-assisted relaxation, can be effective in managing insomnia and stress-related sleep disorders. These approaches focus on training individuals to control physiological responses, reducing tension and promoting relaxation conducive to sleep.

Neurostimulation Therapies: Emerging Approaches for Sleep Apnea

Neurostimulation therapies, including hypoglossal nerve stimulation (HNS) or transcutaneous electrical nerve stimulation (TENS), are emerging as options for managing sleep apnea. These approaches involve stimulating specific nerves or muscles to maintain airway patency during sleep. Neurostimulation therapies are often considered when other treatments, such as CPAP, are not well-tolerated.

As sleep medicine continues to evolve, ongoing research may reveal new and innovative treatment modalities. Tailoring interventions to address the specific characteristics of each sleep disorder ensures a comprehensive and personalised approach to improving sleep quality. Individuals experiencing sleep-related challenges should consult with healthcare professionals to explore the most suitable treatment options based on their unique circumstances.

Quote

"In the quiet shadows of the night, sleep disorders cast intricate patterns on the fabric of rest. Yet, within the labyrinth of challenges, there exists the resilience to unravel complexities, forging a path towards the peaceful serenity that each night deserves."

"In the silent hours of the night, sleep disorders cast shadows on the canvas of rest, yet within the struggle, resilience emerges as the guiding star towards a dawn of renewed tranquility."

One notable figure with a well-documented sleep disorder is Elon Musk. Musk has openly discussed his struggles with insomnia and how it has impacted his work schedule and overall well-being. His candidness about the challenges of managing sleep in a high-demand career sheds light on the importance of addressing sleep disorders and finding effective solutions for optimal health.

Sleep and Productivity

The Productivity Paradox: Sleep as a Cornerstone

In the fast-paced landscape of modern life, there exists a paradoxical relationship between sleep and productivity. While the societal emphasis on productivity often leads to sleep deprivation as individuals extend waking hours to meet demands, this approach can backfire. Sleep is a cornerstone of cognitive functioning, memory consolidation, and overall mental well-being. Prioritising sufficient and quality sleep is not a detractor from productivity; rather, it serves as a catalyst for enhanced cognitive abilities, sharper focus, and improved decision-making.

Cognitive Functioning and Sleep Quality: Partners in Performance

The quality of sleep directly influences cognitive functioning and, consequently, workplace productivity. Sleep is essential for memory consolidation and learning, contributing to improved problem-solving skills and creative thinking.

Individuals who consistently experience restorative sleep are better equipped to handle complex tasks, adapt to changes, and navigate challenges effectively. Furthermore, adequate sleep supports sustained attention, preventing the decline in cognitive performance that often accompanies sleep deprivation.

Mood Regulation: A Sleep-Induced Boost

Emotional well-being is intimately connected to sleep, and mood regulation plays a pivotal role in workplace dynamics. Insufficient sleep is linked to increased irritability, stress, and reduced emotional resilience. Conversely, prioritising restful nights fosters a positive mood and enhances the ability to cope with workplace stressors. A well-rested individual is better positioned to approach tasks with enthusiasm, collaborate effectively with colleagues, and contribute to a positive work environment.

Strategic Napping: A Tactical Approach to Boosting Productivity

Strategic napping emerges as a tactical tool for boosting productivity. Short naps, typically ranging from 10 to 20 minutes, have been shown to improve alertness, mood, and overall performance. Companies recognising the significance of employee well-being have increasingly embraced nap-friendly policies, acknowledging that brief moments of rest can yield substantial gains in focus and productivity. Embracing the symbiotic relationship between sleep and productivity can redefine the workplace narrative, fostering a culture where well-rested individuals contribute to a more innovative, resilient, and high-performing team.

Sleep and Decision-Making: The Cognitive Edge

Sound decision-making is integral to success in any professional setting. Sleep plays a critical role in enhancing cognitive functions, including decision-making abilities. A well-rested mind is better equipped to analyse information, weigh options, and make thoughtful decisions. Conversely, sleep deprivation can impair judgment, increase impulsivity, and lead to suboptimal choices. Recognising the impact of sleep on decision-making underscores the importance of prioritising rest for effective leadership and workplace performance.

Creativity Unleashed: Sleep's Influence on Innovation

Creativity and innovation are essential components of a thriving workplace. Quality sleep has been linked to improved creative thinking and problem-solving skills. During sleep, the brain consolidates memories and reorganises information, fostering connections between seemingly unrelated concepts. This process, known as memory integration, can lead to innovative insights and novel solutions to challenges. Embracing the role of sleep in nurturing creativity positions well-rested individuals as catalysts for innovation within their professional spheres.

Workplace Safety: Sleep as a Risk Mitigator

The impact of sleep extends beyond cognitive functions to encompass physical safety in the workplace. Sleep deprivation is associated with an increased risk of accidents and injuries. In industries that involve complex machinery or require vigilant attention to detail, prioritising adequate sleep is a crucial safety measure. Organisations that recognise the role of sleep-in mitigating workplace risks prioritise employee well-being, fostering a safer and more productive work environment.

Understanding the multifaceted relationship between sleep and productivity allows individuals and organisations to make informed choices that prioritise well-being and optimise performance. By acknowledging sleep as a strategic asset rather than an expendable commodity, workplaces can cultivate a culture that values the health, creativity, and productivity of their teams.

The Foundation of Daytime Performance: Quality Sleep

Quality sleep serves as the bedrock for optimal daytime performance in various facets of life. When individuals consistently experience restful and sufficient sleep, their cognitive functions are sharpened, enhancing memory consolidation, learning, and problem-solving skills. This cognitive resilience forms the basis for improved attention, focus, and overall mental acuity throughout the day.

Recognising the integral role of quality sleep establishes a framework for sustained daytime performance.

Cognitive Functions and Alertness: A Symbiotic Relationship

The symbiotic relationship between quality sleep and cognitive functions directly influences daytime alertness. During sleep, the brain consolidates memories, clears unnecessary information, and prepares for the challenges of the following day. This preparation translates into heightened alertness, ensuring individuals are more responsive to stimuli, better able to process information, and adept at tackling cognitive tasks. Daytime performance is intricately tied to the degree of cognitive alertness maintained through consistent and restorative sleep.

Emotional Regulation: Navigating Day-to-Day Interactions

Quality sleep plays a pivotal role in emotional regulation, influencing how individuals navigate day-to-day interactions and manage stressors. Adequate sleep fosters emotional resilience, enabling individuals to respond more effectively to challenges and fluctuations in mood. Conversely, sleep deprivation can contribute to heightened emotional reactivity, increased irritability, and difficulty managing stress. A well-rested individual is better equipped to maintain emotional equilibrium, fostering positive interactions and enhancing overall interpersonal dynamics.

Physical Vitality: Energising the Body for Daily Demands

Beyond cognitive and emotional aspects, quality sleep is crucial for physical vitality, providing the energy needed to meet the demands of daily life. The restoration and repair processes that occur during sleep contribute to overall physical well-being. This vitality, in turn, supports engagement in physical activities, sustains stamina throughout the day, and aids in the prevention of fatigue. Recognising the link between quality sleep and physical vitality underscores the importance of prioritising rest as an essential component of a healthy and high-performing lifestyle.

Strategies for improving work efficiency.

Time Management Mastery: Prioritising Tasks

Effective time management is a cornerstone of work efficiency. Prioritise tasks based on urgency and importance, utilising techniques such as the Eisenhower Matrix to categorise responsibilities. By focusing on high-priority tasks first, you ensure that critical objectives are addressed promptly, enhancing overall work efficiency. Implementing time-blocking strategies, where specific periods are dedicated to particular tasks, further streamlines daily workflows, minimising distractions and optimising productivity.

Goal Setting and Planning: Roadmaps to Success

Setting clear goals and creating actionable plans provide a roadmap to success. Break down larger projects into smaller, manageable tasks, setting realistic deadlines for each. This approach not only enhances clarity but also fosters a sense of accomplishment as milestones are achieved. Regularly revisit and adjust goals as needed, ensuring they align with broader objectives. A well-defined plan instills focus, aiding in the efficient allocation of time and resources toward goal attainment.

Streamlining Communication: Efficient Collaboration

Effective communication is essential for workplace efficiency. Implement streamlined communication channels, utilising tools such as project management platforms, instant messaging, or collaborative documents. Clearly define roles and expectations, ensuring that team members are on the same page. Regular check-ins and status updates minimise misunderstandings and facilitate a smooth flow of information, contributing to cohesive teamwork and efficient project execution.

Embracing Technology: Automation and Integration

Leveraging technology can significantly enhance work efficiency. Identify tasks that can be automated, reducing manual workload and minimising errors. Integration of software tools, from project management systems to communication platforms, fosters seamless workflows. Stay abreast of emerging technologies relevant to your industry, exploring how they can be harnessed to streamline processes and elevate overall work efficiency.

Continuous Learning and Skill Development: Staying Relevant

Investing in continuous learning and skill development ensures that you stay relevant and proficient in your role. Acquiring new skills not only enhances your individual capabilities but can also introduce innovative approaches to tasks. Attend workshops, enrol in online courses, or seek mentorship opportunities to expand your skill set. The ability to adapt and acquire new knowledge positions you as an invaluable asset within your organisation, contributing to heightened work efficiency.

Strategic Breaks and Mindful Rest: Sustaining Productivity

Recognise the importance of strategic breaks and mindful rest in sustaining productivity. Implement the Comodoro Technique or similar methods, incorporating short breaks between focused work intervals. Physical activity during breaks can boost energy levels and enhance cognitive function. Ensure that longer breaks allow for genuine relaxation, aiding in stress reduction and preventing burnout. Prioritising both focused work and intentional rest contributes to sustained work efficiency and overall well-being.

Cultivating a mindful sleep mindset

Cultivating a mindset for sleep involves shaping your thoughts and beliefs around the concept of sleep. It's about adopting a mental framework that values and priorities rest. This mindset may include recognising the importance of sleep for overall well-being, acknowledging the significance of a consistent sleep schedule, and understanding the connection between mental health and quality sleep. In essence, it's the psychological foundation that influences your approach to sleep.

On the other hand, developing positive habits for sleep involves creating intentional and constructive behaviours that contribute to a conducive sleep environment. These habits can encompass a range of activities, such as establishing a regular bedtime routine, creating a comfortable sleep environment, limiting screen time before bed, and engaging in relaxation techniques. Positive sleep habits are the actionable steps you take to support and enhance the quality of your sleep.

While cultivating a mindset for sleep sets the stage by influencing your beliefs and attitudes, developing positive habits for sleep translates those thoughts into tangible, daily practices. Both elements work synergistically – a positive mindset can motivate the adoption of healthy sleep habits, and engaging in positive habits reinforces and strengthens the sleep-supportive mindset. Together, they form a comprehensive approach to fostering a restful and rejuvenating sleep experience.

Creating a Relaxing Bedtime Routine: A Prelude to Sleep

Cultivating a mindful sleep mindset begins with establishing a relaxing bedtime routine. Create a calming pre-sleep ritual that signals to your body and mind that it's time to wind down. This may include activities such as reading a book, practicing gentle stretching or yoga, or engaging in mindfulness meditation. Consistency is key in reinforcing the association between these calming activities and the transition to sleep.

Digital Detox: Unplugging for Tranquility

Mindful sleep involves disconnecting from the digital world before bedtime. The blue light emitted by screens can disrupt the production of melatonin, a hormone essential for sleep. Establish a digital detox routine by powering down electronic devices at least an hour before bed. Consider replacing screen time with activities that promote relaxation and tranquility, setting the stage for a more restful sleep experience.

Thought Awareness: Managing Mental Chatter

A mindful sleep mindset involves managing mental chatter and reducing the impact of racing thoughts. Practice thought awareness by acknowledging any worries or thoughts that arise, but gently redirect your focus to the present moment. Techniques such as journaling before bedtime or engaging in a brief mindfulness meditation can help calm the mind and release mental tension, creating a conducive mental environment for sleep.

Gratitude Practice: Shifting Focus to Positivity

Incorporating a gratitude practice before bedtime can shift your focus from stressors to positive aspects of your day. Reflect on moments of gratitude, whether big or small, fostering a sense of contentment. This practice not only enhances overall well-being but also promotes a more positive mindset as you approach sleep. Gratitude journaling or simply mentally noting a few things you're thankful for can become a powerful bedtime ritual.

Creating a Comfortable Sleep Environment: Mindful Rest

Mindful sleep extends to the physical space where you rest. Evaluate and optimise your sleep environment to enhance comfort and tranquility. This may involve adjusting room temperature, investing in a comfortable mattress and pillows, and minimising noise and light disturbances. Creating a serene sleep environment signal to your body that it's a safe and peaceful space for restorative sleep.

Breathing Techniques: Calming the Nervous System

Mindful breathing techniques can be instrumental in calming the nervous system and promoting relaxation. Consider incorporating deep breathing exercises or guided breathing meditations before bedtime. Focus on slow, rhythmic breaths to activate the body's relaxation response. This mindful approach to breathing not only facilitates a smoother transition to sleep but also cultivates a sense of mindfulness that can extend into other areas of your life.

Mindful Nutrition: Evening Nourishment

Mindful sleep extends to mindful nutrition. Be conscious of your evening food choices, opting for a light and balanced meal. Avoid heavy or caffeine-laden foods close to bedtime, as they can disrupt sleep. Consider incorporating sleep-inducing foods that contain tryptophan, such as turkey, dairy, or nuts. Being mindful of your evening nutrition supports your body's natural sleep processes.

Progressive Muscle Relaxation: Physical Unwinding

Progressive muscle relaxation (PMR) is a mindfulness technique that involves systematically tensing and then relaxing different muscle groups. This practice helps release physical tension and promotes overall relaxation. Incorporate PMR into your bedtime routine, progressively moving through your body to release tension. This physical unwinding contributes to a state of calmness, facilitating the transition into a more restful sleep.

Cultivating a mindful sleep mindset involves a holistic approach that encompasses various aspects of your evening routine, environment, and mental state. Experiment with different mindfulness practices to discover what resonates most with you, and tailor them to create a personalised bedtime ritual. By consistently embracing these mindful practices, you can foster a deep sense of relaxation and contribute to a more peaceful and rejuvenating sleep experience.

Quote

"In the stillness before slumber, cultivate a mindful sleep mindset – where each breath becomes a lullaby, and the quietude of the mind invites dreams to dance freely, creating a sanctuary for restful serenity."

Michelle Obama, former First Lady of the United States, has emphasised the significance of sleep in maintaining a healthy lifestyle. She has spoken about prioritising sleep for physical and mental well-being. Obama's sleep mindset revolves around self-care, recognising that a good night's sleep is essential for resilience and navigating the demands of a busy life with grace and vitality.

Mindfulness and its impact on sleep

Mindfulness, when applied to sleep and sleeping habits, involves cultivating a heightened awareness and presence in the present moment. The impact of mindfulness on sleep is often twofold, addressing both the mental aspects of sleep quality and the habits that influence our nightly routines.

In terms of sleep quality, mindfulness practices such as meditation and deep-breathing exercises can help calm the mind, reduce stress, and alleviate anxiety that may be contributing to sleep disturbances. By fostering a state of relaxation and promoting a more restful mental space, mindfulness contributes to improved sleep patterns.

On the other hand, when considering sleeping habits, mindfulness can play a crucial role in shaping our routines. It encourages individuals to be present and intentional in their actions, from winding down before bedtime to creating a tranquil sleep environment. Mindful sleep habits may involve disconnecting from screens, establishing a consistent bedtime routine, and being aware of the impact of lifestyle choices on sleep, such as diet and exercise.

In summary, the impact of mindfulness on sleep is comprehensive. It addresses both the mental and behavioural aspects of sleep, fostering a holistic approach to improving sleep quality and establishing healthy sleeping habits.

Understanding Mindfulness: Present-Moment Awareness

Mindfulness, rooted in ancient contemplative practices, involves cultivating present-moment awareness without judgment. In the context of sleep, mindfulness is about being fully present in the moments leading up to bedtime and during the sleep process itself. It encourages individuals to acknowledge thoughts, feelings, and sensations without becoming entangled in them. This non-judgmental awareness lays the foundation for a more tranquil and focused approach to sleep.

Reducing Stress and Anxiety: A Gateway to Better Sleep

One of the significant impacts of mindfulness on sleep is its ability to alleviate stress and anxiety. Mindfulness practices, such as mindfulness meditation or mindful breathing, activate the body's relaxation response. By shifting attention away from future concerns or past events, individuals can create a mental space that promotes tranquility. This reduction in stress and anxiety levels can be particularly beneficial for those who struggle with racing thoughts or insomnia, contributing to an improved sleep environment.

Improving Sleep Quality: Enhancing Sleep Architecture

Mindfulness has been associated with improvements in sleep quality and sleep architecture. Regular mindfulness practices have shown positive effects on sleep continuity, the proportion of time spent in restorative sleep stages, and overall sleep efficiency. Mindfulness meditation, for example, can positively influence the release of sleep-regulating hormones and neurotransmitters, promoting a more robust and rejuvenating sleep experience.

Managing Sleep Disorders: Mindfulness-Based Interventions

Mindfulness-based interventions, such as Mindfulness-Based Stress Reduction (MBSR) or Mindfulness-Based Cognitive Therapy (MBCT), have been increasingly incorporated into the treatment of sleep disorders. These structured programs blend mindfulness practices with cognitive-behavioural strategies to address underlying factors contributing to sleep challenges. Participants learn to cultivate mindful awareness, manage stressors, and develop healthier sleep habits, leading to sustained improvements in sleep quality.

Enhancing Sleep Mindset: A Holistic Approach

Beyond specific techniques, mindfulness contributes to a more holistic sleep mindset. It encourages a compassionate attitude towards oneself, acknowledging that sleep is a natural process influenced by various factors. This mindset shift helps individuals let go of perfectionistic expectations about sleep, reducing performance anxiety related to bedtime. By embracing a mindful approach, individuals can create a positive and accepting attitude towards sleep, fostering an environment conducive to restful nights and overall well-being.:

Mindful Breathing and Relaxation: Calming the Nervous System

Mindful breathing techniques play a crucial role in calming the nervous system and preparing the body for sleep. Practices such as deep belly breathing or diaphragmatic breathing can activate the parasympathetic nervous system, often referred to as the "rest and digest" system. By consciously regulating the breath, individuals can reduce physiological arousal, lower heart rate, and create a sense of calm conducive to the onset of sleep.

Mindfulness-Based Stress Reduction (MBSR): A Comprehensive Approach

Mindfulness-Based Stress Reduction (MBSR) is a structured program that incorporates mindfulness meditation and yoga to promote overall well-being, including improved sleep. MBSR teaches individuals to cultivate awareness in their daily lives, manage stress more effectively, and develop a healthier relationship with their thoughts and emotions. As stress reduction is a key component, participants often report enhanced sleep quality as a natural byproduct of the program.

Mindful Movement: Yoga and Sleep Connection

Mindful movement practices, particularly yoga, offer a unique synergy with sleep. Gentle yoga poses, combined with mindful awareness of breath and body sensations, create a mindful movement experience. This combination of physical activity and mindfulness can help release tension, improve flexibility, and promote relaxation, contributing to better sleep quality. Evening yoga routines specifically designed for sleep often incorporate poses and sequences conducive to winding down and preparing the body for rest.

Mindfulness Apps for Sleep: Integrating Technology Mindfully

In the digital age, mindfulness apps tailored for sleep have gained popularity. These apps often feature guided meditations, calming sounds, or bedtime stories designed to promote relaxation and mindfulness. While integrating technology into the bedtime routine requires a mindful approach, these apps can serve as accessible tools for individuals looking to infuse mindfulness practices into their sleep preparation.

Long-Term Mindfulness Practices: Building Resilience

Engaging in mindfulness practices over the long term contributes to building emotional resilience and adaptability. By developing a heightened awareness of the present moment, individuals may find it easier to navigate life's challenges and uncertainties. This increased resilience can extend to how individuals cope with stressors that may impact their sleep, fostering a more sustainable and positive relationship with the sleep experience over time.

Quote

"In the embrace of bedtime, let mindfulness be the
gentle conductor of your dreams – weaving each
breath into a serene melody, guiding you through the
peaceful landscapes of a mindful sleep."

"As night unfolds its silent symphony, practice
mindfulness in the realm of sleep – let each
conscious breath be a calming breeze, and watch
tranquility bloom in the gardens of your dreams."

Developing Healthy sleep habits

Consistent Sleep Schedule: Setting Circadian Rhythms

Establishing a consistent sleep schedule is foundational to developing healthy sleep habits. Aim to go to bed and wake up at the same time every day, even on weekends. This regularity helps set and reinforce circadian rhythms, the body's internal clock, promoting better sleep quality and overall sleep-wake consistency. Consistency in sleep patterns contributes to improved energy levels, mood, and cognitive function.

Create a Relaxing Bedtime Routine: Unwind Before Sleep

Crafting a calming bedtime routine signals to the body that it's time to wind down and prepare for sleep. Engage in activities that promote relaxation, such as reading a book, taking a warm bath, or practicing gentle stretches. Consistency in your bedtime routine helps cue the body that sleep is imminent, enhancing the ease with which you transition into restful slumber.

Mindful Use of Electronics: Limiting Screen Time

Mindful use of electronics is crucial for healthy sleep habits. The blue light emitted by screens can suppress the production of melatonin, a hormone that regulates sleep. Aim to power down electronic devices at least an hour before bedtime. Consider replacing screen time with activities that support relaxation, such as listening to calming music or practicing mindfulness meditation. This mindful approach helps create an environment conducive to restful sleep.

Optimise Sleep Environment: Create a Sleep Sanctuary

Crafting an optimal sleep environment contributes to healthy sleep habits. Ensure your bedroom is cool, dark, and quiet. Invest in a comfortable mattress and pillows that provide proper support. Minimise noise and light disturbances to create a sleep sanctuary that promotes restful nights. Keeping the bedroom dedicated primarily to sleep enhances the association between the sleep environment and rest, reinforcing healthy sleep habits.

Limit Caffeine and Nicotine Intake: Mindful Consumption

The mindful consumption of stimulants like caffeine and nicotine plays a significant role in healthy sleep habits. Avoid consuming these substances, especially in the hours leading up to bedtime, as they can interfere with the ability to fall asleep and reduce overall sleep quality. Be mindful of hidden sources of caffeine, such as certain medications or chocolate, and aim to limit intake for a smoother transition into restorative sleep.

Regular Physical Activity: Energising the Body for Sleep

Incorporating regular physical activity into your routine supports healthy sleep habits. Engage in moderate exercise, such as brisk walking or yoga, on a regular basis. However, avoid vigorous exercise close to bedtime, as it may have a stimulating effect.

Physical activity helps expend energy, reduces stress, and contributes to a more restful sleep experience. Mindfully integrating exercise into your daily life supports overall well-being and enhances the foundation for healthy sleep habits.

Conclusion

In Closing: Embracing the Journey to Better Sleep

As we conclude this exploration of the intricate world of sleep, it's essential to reflect on the transformative power of cultivating healthy sleep habits. Sleep is not merely a biological necessity but a cornerstone of well-being that permeates every facet of our lives. The journey to better sleep is a personal odyssey, a quest to unlock the potential for restorative rest and awaken a more vibrant, resilient self.

Acknowledging the Importance of Mindfulness

Mindfulness emerges as a guiding principle throughout this journey. From mindful bedtime routines to the practice of gratitude and the art of mindful breathing, each chapter underscores the profound impact of cultivating present-moment awareness on our sleep and, by extension, our overall quality of life. Mindfulness becomes a trusted companion, offering solace in the tranquility of the present moment and infusing our nights with a sense of peaceful surrender.

Building Bridges Between Science and Practical Tips

The pages of this book have sought to bridge the realms of scientific understanding and practical strategies. We've delved into the stages of sleep, the intricacies of circadian rhythms, and the profound effects of sleep on our physical and mental health. Woven through these insights are actionable tips and strategies—practical tools designed to empower you on your quest for better sleep. These bridges connect the theoretical with the tangible, providing a roadmap for translating knowledge into transformative habits.

The Interconnected Nature of Sleep and Well-Being

Sleep, we've discovered, is not a solitary act but part of a symphony of factors influencing our well-being. From the quality of our daily routines to the depth of our emotional resilience, the threads of sleep are interwoven with the fabric of our lives. By embracing the interconnected nature of sleep and well-being, we embark on a holistic approach that nurtures not only our nights but also our waking hours, fostering a more vibrant and fulfilling existence.

Nurturing a Mindful Sleep Mindset

At the heart of this journey is the cultivation of a mindful sleep mindset. Mindfulness becomes a lantern guiding us through the quiet moments before sleep, the challenges of daily life, and the spaces where dreams unfold. It's an invitation to savour the beauty of rest, to be present in the nocturnal embrace, and to approach sleep with a sense of reverence. In nurturing a mindful sleep mindset, we unlock the door to a sanctuary where rest and wakefulness coexist harmoniously.

Embrace the Progress, No Matter How Small

Embarking on the journey to better sleep is an empowering decision, and it's crucial to recognise and celebrate every step forward, no matter how small. Progress in cultivating healthy sleep habits may not happen overnight, and that's perfectly okay. Each mindful choice, whether it's creating a soothing bedtime routine or prioritising consistent sleep schedules, contributes to the gradual transformation of your sleep landscape. Embrace the journey with patience and self-compassion, knowing that positive changes are unfolding, one night at a time.

You Have the Power to Redefine Your Relationship with Sleep

Remember that you hold the power to redefine your relationship with sleep. It's not about perfection, but about embracing the opportunities to enhance your well-being through conscious choices. By acknowledging the importance of sleep and approaching it with a mindful mindset, you're laying the groundwork for a healthier, more balanced life. Trust in your ability to shape your sleep habits and, in turn, positively influence your physical, mental, and emotional vitality.

Every Night Is a Fresh Start

As you navigate the twists and turns of the sleep journey, keep in mind that every night is a fresh start. Regardless of the challenges faced or setbacks encountered, each new evening presents an opportunity to recalibrate and recommit to your goals. Allow yourself the grace to learn from experiences, adjust your strategies, and move forward with renewed determination. With each sunset, you embark on a new chapter in the story of

your sleep journey—one where the promise of rest
and rejuvenation awaits.

A Continuation of the Sleep Odyssey

As we bid farewell to these pages, the journey to better sleep continues. It's a journey of discovery, of listening to the whispers of our bodies and the rhythms of the night. The chapters may end, but the odyssey persists in the choices we make, the habits we cultivate, and the mindfulness we bring to each sleep-filled moment. May your nights be restful, your dreams be sweet, and your waking hours be infused with the vitality that comes from honouring the profound importance of sleep in the tapestry of life.

Thank you

Thank you, dear reader, for embarking on this exploration of sleep, its challenges, and the avenues towards improvement. Your time and attention are deeply appreciated. As you navigate the pages, may you find insights that resonate with your own sleep journey, and perhaps discover strategies to enhance the quality of your rest. In the quiet moments between these words, I hope you uncover valuable nuggets of wisdom that lead to peaceful nights and rejuvenated mornings. May this journey through the realms of sleep be a catalyst for positive changes in your well-being, and may the nights ahead bring you the restful embrace you truly deserve.

Final quote

"Embark on the nocturnal odyssey of self-care, where each mindful step and tranquil breath pave the way to a sanctuary of better sleep. In the realm of the night, may your journey be guided by the wisdom of rest, unlocking the transformative power of sleep for a brighter, more rejuvenated life."